# ECHINACEA

Woodland Publishing
*Pleasant Grove, UT*

# TABLE OF CONTENTS

# ECHINACEA

## (*Echinacea angustifolia*)

*Common Names:* Black Sampson, purple coneflower, rudbeckia, Missouri snakeroot, red sunflower

*Plant Parts:* roots, rhizome

*Active Compounds:* echinacoside, polysaccharides (echinacin), antibiotic polyacetylenes, betaine, caffeic acid glycosides, inulin, isobutyl amides, essential oil (humulene, caryophylene), isobutyl-alkylamines, resin, flavonoids (in leaves and stems), sesquiterpene esters (echinadiole, epoxy-echinadiole, echinax-anthole, and dihydor-xynardole)

*Pharmacology:* Echinacea contains a variety of chemical compounds that have significant pharmacological functions. It has been the subject of hundreds of clinical and scientific studies which have primarily used an extract of the plant portion of the botanical. The rich content of polysaccharides and phytosterols in echinacea are what make it a strong immune system stimulant. The sesquiterpene esters also have immunostimulatory effects. Glycoside echinacoside is found in the roots of the plant. Echinacin has also been found to possess anti-fungal and antibiotic properties. This component of echinacea also has cortisone-like actions which can help promote the healing of wounds and helps to control the inflammatory reactions of allergies.

*Vitamin and Mineral Content:* vitamins A, E, C, iron, iodine, copper, sulphur and potassium

*Character:* alterative, antibiotic, antiseptic, antiviral, anti-inflammatory, immuno-stimulant, carminative, depurgative, fermentative, demulcent, lymphatic tonic, and vulnerary

*Body Systems Targeted:* immune system, lymph system, blood and kidneys

## Herbal Forms

*Decoction:* A tea or decoction made from echinacea is good for the acute stage of any infection.

*Tincture:* This form of echinacea is also effective for infections such as influenza, urinary tract, glandular fever etc. Echinacea tinctures have be used in concentrated form for food poisoning and snakebite.

*Wash:* Can be used as a decoction or diluted tincture for infected wounds.

*Ointment:* Can be used for direct application on burns or other skin wounds.

*Powder:* Can be dusted on infected skin conditions such as boils or eczema.

*Capsules:* Echinacea capsules are used for acute infections such as colds, flu, urinary tract or kidney infections.

*Gargle:* Echinacea tincture can be combined with water to make a gargle for sore throats.

*Fresh Pressed Juice:* Some commercial preparations offer this form; however, because it requires a freshly harvested plant, it may be more difficult to obtain.

*Storage:* Keep in a cool, dry environment.

*Regulatory Status*

| | |
|---|---|
| U.S.: | None |
| U.K.: | General sales list |
| Canada: | Over-the-counter drug status |
| France: | None |
| Germany: | Commission E approved as drug |

*Recommended Usage:* Echinacea works best if it is taken right at the onset of an infection in substantial doses and then tapered off. It can be used in higher quantities as a preventative during winter months when colds and flu are prevalent. If using it to maintain the immune system, periodic use is believed to be more effective than continual usage. Typically, one should use echinacea for seven to eight weeks followed by one week off. Guaranteed potency echinacea is currently available in capsule form only.

*Safety:* High doses can occasionally cause nausea and dizziness. Echinacea has not exhibited any observed toxicity even in high dosages. Anyone who is suffering from any type of kidney disorder should restrict taking echinacea to one week maximum. Very heavy use of echinacea may temporarily cause male infertility.

# HISTORY

Because 20th-century medical practices have routinely over-prescribed antibiotics, the notion of a natural antibiotic with virtually no side-effects is intriguing to say the least. Echinacea is one of several herbs which possesses antibacterial, antiviral and antifungal properties. In a time when new life-threatening microbes are evolving and pose the threat of modern-day plagues, herbs such as echinacea are particularly valuable. More and more health practitioners are focusing on fortifying the immune system to fight off potential infections rather than just treating infection after it has developed.

Echinacea is enjoying a renaissance today. During the late 1980s, echinacea re-emerged as a remarkable medicinal plant. In addition to its infection fighting properties, echinacea is known for its healing properties as well. As was the case with so many herbs, echinacea lost its prestige as a medicinal treatment with the advent of antibiotics. It has experienced a resurgence over the last two decades.

Echinacea has several other much more romantic names including purple coneflower, Black Sampson and red sunflower. It has also become the common name for a number of echinacea species like E. angustifolia, E. purpurea, and E. pallida. The genus derives its name from the Greek word *echinos* which refers to sea urchin. This particular association evolved from the prickly spiny scales of the seed head section of the flower. Historically, echinacea has sometimes become confused with *Parthenium integrifolium*.

The word echinacea is actually a part of the scientific latin term, *echinacea angustifolia,* which literally translated means a narrow-leafed sucker. The plant grows wild as a perennial exclusively in the midwestern plains states, but can be cultivated almost anywhere. Echinacea leaves are pale to dark green, coarse and pointy. Its florets are purple, and its roots are black and long.

Echinacea has a strong Native American link in the central plains. Native Americans are credited with discovering the usefulness of this botanical without knowing its specific chemical properties. It was routinely used by Native Americans to treat toothaches, snakebite, fevers and old stubborn wounds.

Native Americans thought of echinacea as a versatile herb that not only helped to fight infection, but increased the appetite and strengthened the sexual organs as well. The juice of the plant was used to bathe burns and was sprinkled on hot coals during traditional "sweats" used for purification purposes. It is also believed that some Native Americans used echinacea juice to protect their hands, feet and mouths from the heat of hot coals and ceremonial fires.[1]

According to Melvin Gilmore, an American anthropologist who studied Native American medicine in the early part of this century, echinacea was used as a remedy by Native Americans more than any other plant in the central plains area.[2]

In time, early white settlers learned of its healing powers and used the plant as a home remedy for colds, influenza, tumors, syphillis, hemorrhoids and wounds. Dr. John King, in his medical journal of 1887, mentioned that echinacea had value as a blood purifier and alterative. It was used in various blood tonics and gained the reputation of being good for almost every conceivable malady. It has been called the king of blood purifiers due to its ability to improve lymphatic filtration and drainage. In time, echinacea became popular with 19th-century Eclectics, who were followers of a botanic system founded by Dr. Wooster Beech in the 1830s. They used it as an anesthetic, deodorant, and stimulant.

By 1898, echinacea had become one of the top natural treatments in America. During these years, echinacea was used to treat fevers, malignant carbuncles, ulcerations, pyorrhea, snake bites and dermatitis. In the early twentieth century, echinacea had gained a formidable reputation for treating a long list of infectious disease ranging from the commonplace to the exotic. The Lloyd Brothers Pharmaceutical House developed more sophisticated versions of the herb in order to meet escalating demands for echinacea.

Ironically, it was medical doctors who considered echinacea more valuable than eclectic practitioners. Several articles on echinacea appeared from time to time in various publications. Its attributes were reviewed and, at times, its curative abilities ranged from the sublime to the ridiculous. In 1909, the Council on Pharmacy and Chemistry of the American Medical Association decided against recognizing echinacea as an official drug, claiming that it lacked scientific credibility. It was added to the National Formulary of the United States despite this type of negative reaction and remained on this list until 1950.

Over the past 50 years, echinacea has earned a formidable reputation achieving worldwide fame for its antiviral, antifungal and antibacterial actions. Consumer interest in echinacea has greatly increased, particularly in relation to its role in treating candida, chronic fatigue syndrome, AIDS and malignancies. Practitioners of natural medicine in Europe and America have long valued its attributes. In recent, years, German research has confirmed its ability to augment the human immune system. Extensive research on echinacea has occurred over the last twenty years. Test results have shown that the herb has an antibiotic, cortisone-like activity. Echinacea has the ability to boost cell membrane healing, protect collagen, and suppress tumor growth.

Because of its immuno-enhancing activity, it has recently been used in AIDS therapy. Research has proven that echinacea may have profound value in stimulating immune function and may be particularly beneficial for colds and sore throats.[3]

# FUNCTIONS

Echinacea increases the body's ability to resist and fight infection, clears the blood of impurities and has been used for fevers, venereal diseases, hemorrhoids and as an aphrodisiac. Unquestionably, its most important function as a botanical is as an immune system booster and blood purifier. For this reason, it has recently been considered for AIDS therapy.

Echinacea is one of the most useful herbs available to practitioners because it functions to simultaneously stimulate the immune system, while it expedites the removal of toxins from the body.

Echinacea is recommended for common infections and can be tried in lieu of or in combination with conventional antibiotics.[4] It is better to take the herb for two weeks at a time alternating with two weeks off to ensure its efficacy.

It is an effective therapeutic agent for healing wounds, treating abscesses, carbuncles, eczema, burns, psoriasis, herpes, canker sores, typhoid fever, viral and bacterial infections and tumors.

# Blood Purifier

Echinacea is considered one of the best blood purifiers found in nature. It has been scientifically researched for its chemical ability to neutralize harmful venom from poisonous snakes, scorpions, insects and other toxic substances. Laboratory tests have found that certain complex chemicals found in echinacea have the ability to rearrange and recognize enzyme patterns in the body.[5] It also improves lymphatic filtration and drainage and assists in clearing the blood from damaging toxins. It has traditionally been referred to as the "king of the blood purifiers."

Any condition which is believed to be caused by an accumulation of toxins in the body can benefit from echinacea.

# Immune System Booster

In 1885, Rudolf Weiss recorded, "It [echinacea] has proved a useful drug in improving the body's own resistance in infectious conditions of all kind."[6] Clearly, echinacea has potent immune system actions and impacts the thymus gland, the activation of T-cells, and the promotion of interferon production and secretion. Because of these attributes, it is an important herb in combating infections, especially viral ones like AIDS and chronic fatigue syndrome.

The major component of echinacea, called inulin, is responsible for activating pathways in the body, which help neutralize viruses and bacteria, and boost the migration of white blood cells to infection sites. The natural polysaccharides, fatty acids and glycosides in this botanical all strengthen and nourish the immune system. Echinacea is considered an immuno-tonic, which supplies the immune system with specific nutrients.

Echinacea has the capability to stimulate the immune response which results in an increased ability to resist infections. It is the most widely used herb for the enhancement of the immune system and is valuable for treating virtually all infectious diseases. Studies have shown that echinacea has impressive immune system boosting properties, many of which are produced in the thymus gland.[7]

One way in which echinacea helps the body combat infection is by enhancing the immune function of white blood cells. In order for white blood cells to effectively fight bacterial or viral invasion, nutrients such as vitamin A, vitamin C and zinc are necessary. Adding echinacea potentiates any nutrient mix, which helps facilitate the production of white blood cells. White blood cells surround and destroy bacterial and viral invaders. Technically, they digest disease organisms; a process called phagocytosis. Echinacea makes phagocytosis more efficient. The white blood cells which participate in phagocytosis are called macrophages. In several laboratory studies, echinacea has repeatedly stimulated the bactericide activity of macrophages. In other words, it potentiates their ability to destroy invading organisms.

## Echinacea, Radiation and Chemotherapy

For anyone who has to undergo radiation treatments, echinacea can also be beneficial. One of the drawbacks of both radiation and chemotherapy is that white blood cells are destroyed by the treatments. The particular therapeutic action of echinacea discussed above shows that it can stimulate an increase in white blood cells following radiation treatments. These findings also suggest that echinacea works best if taken early, before the infection spreads. In light of these studies, taking echinacea is recommended for those undergoing cancer radiation or chemotherapy.

## The Dual Immune Function of Echinacea

What is fascinating about echinacea is that while it can raise white blood cell activity it can also lower it when appropriate. This plant has the ability to affect opposite reactions in the body, and it is the body's condition which determines they type of action initiated. There are no known synthetic drugs which have this dualism to both augment and suppress the immune response according to need.

Laboratory tests have shown that echinacea does, in fact, boost the production of antibodies and T-cells. In the case of any infection, the sooner treatment is started, the better the results will be.

## Interferon Production, T-Lymphocytes, and Echinacea

Interferon is produced in the body primarily by T-cells. The chemical components of interferon are extremely important in activating white blood cells to destroy cancer cells and viruses. Several nutrients can help boost the production of interferon but none seem to have the potency of echinacea. The effect of echinacea is considered remarkable in its ability to stimulate the production and action of interferon.[8] It is this effect which results in significant antiviral actions

T-Lymphocytes are responsible for what is called cell-mediated immunity. In other words, immune functions that are not controlled by antibodies. This type of immunity is vital in protecting the body against certain diseases caused by fungi (such as yeast infections), parasites, moldlike bacteria and viruses. Contracting these types of infections may indicate that the immune system has already been compromised and is susceptible to invasion.

In addition to the disorders listed above, cell-mediated immunity also helps to protect us from autoimmune diseases such as arthritis, allergies and the formation of malignancies.

Interferon is produced by T-Cells and acts to boost and potentiate the immune system. Laboratory tests have confirmed that extracts of the echinacea root contain interferon-like properties.[9] Clearly, interferon boosts immune function and is currently being tested for its potential value in treating cancer. It is produced naturally in the body and enables body systems to resist viral invasion. Some studies have suggested that echinacea may be effective in fighting tumor related and infectious diseases.[10]

Echinacea has been found to effectively prevent the spread of infection.[11] It inhibits the production the action of hyaluronidase, an enzyme which is secreted by invading organisms to make surrounding tissue more susceptible to infection proliferation. Hyaluronic acid is the stuff that glues cells together to create tissue. It is vital to protecting our cell walls against the threat of invasion by disease microbes like strep and staph bacteria. Hyaluronidase breaks down the viscosity of this acid making it possible for organisms to enter and destroy.

In addition, the polysaccharide contained in the herb can protect cells against diseases such as herpes, canker sores, colds, flu and a variety of infections.

# The Lymph System and Echinacea

Echinacea acts as a natural antibiotic and helps to clear toxins from the glands and lymphatic systems. Lymphatic circulation is vital to the immune system. The lymph system is considered the second circulatory system of the body. It cleans the body of excess waste from cellular functions which is discarded through the kidneys.

Lymphatic function can be improved by increasing the circulation of lymph fluid. Echinacea can accomplish this, and in addition, helps to expedite waste products through the lymph system.[12] Apparently, echinacea improves the circulation of both blood and lymph, which can facilitate the removal of waste through the skin, kidneys and the bowel.

# What Infections Respond to Echinacea?

Echinacea extracts are excellent when used for various kinds of acute infections. Colds and throat infections seem particularly vulnerable to the immunostimulant action of echinacea. Infections such as influenza and strep are also affected by the herb.

Again, taking echinacea on a regular basis does not guarantee that the body will not develop an infection; however, the duration and seriousness of the infection should be decreased.

*Antibacterial Action of Echinacea:* It is interesting to note that echinacea renders a mild effect on bacteria. It must be remembered, however, that the ability of echinacea to stimulate the immune system may explain its long historical use for bacterial infections. The echinacoside and caffeic acid content of echinacea have been found to inhibit the growth of bacteria such as *Staphylococcus aureus, Corynebacterium diphtheria* and *Proteus vulgaris.*[13]

*Viral Infections and Echinacea:* Viral infections are notoriously difficult to treat. Even with all the strides that medical technology has made, finding a cure for viral disease has remained elusive. Echinacea stands out as one of the more effective antiviral herbals. The plant has undergone several studies to determine what exactly makes it an effective virus fighter. Several studies have confirmed that when certain laboratory samples were pre-treated with echinacea compounds, they became protected against exposure to several viruses including: influenza, herpes and vesicular stomatitis (canker sores).

Scientists believe that the polysaccharides contained in echinacea called inulin are primarily responsible for the immuno-stimulant effect of this herb. The following listed actions make echinacea especially effective in fighting viral infections and cancerous conditions.

- Promotes macrophage activity
- Stimulates T-cell production
- Stimulates interferon production
- Increases phagocytosis[14]

It is echinacea's ability to stimulate T-cell activity, which subsequently produces interferon, that may be responsible for its anti-viral effect. While this theory has been disputed, ingesting certain forms of echinacea has resulted in some degree of protection against viral infection. Fresh echinacea juice appears to be the most effective form of the herb.

In any case, research strongly suggests than anyone who consumes echinacea regularly can expect protection against some viral infections to a certain degree.

*Respiratory System Infections and Echinacea:* Echinacea has become well known for its ability to treat respiratory infections including influenza, tonsillitis, whooping cough, and colds. In addition, bronchial and ear infections respond well to echinacea therapy. The majority of research that supports this action of echinacea was done in Europe with injectable forms of echinacea which are not legal here.

Using whole, powdered, capsulized echinacea on a daily basis during the winter months may also provide significant protection against these respiratory diseases. Concentrated liquid extract is also recommended.

# Cancer and Echinacea

Some experts believe that over the last 40 years, science has lost its battle with cancer. Progress has been slow and cancer mortality rates continue to rise despite the enormous amount of money spent on research. While most of us are aware of potential carcinogens that surround us, most of us do not take a preventative approach.

In other words, even if we eat nutritiously and try to protect ourselves from toxin exposure, cancers still develop. The role of the immune system in cancer prevention is significant to say the least. Why some people develop cancerous tumors and others do not may be linked to immune function.

We're all aware of the new emphasis on antioxidants today. Likewise, stimulating and strengthening the immune system may also provide significant protection against certain types of malignancy. It's time to concentrate on why some of us don't get cancer instead of focusing all our attention on why some of us do.

In addition to boosting the immune system, echinacea has been shown to increase properdin levels in the body which may be responsible for its anti-cancer activity. By increasing the production and secretion of interferon, echinacea may help enable the body to neutralize carcinogens.[15]

USDA researchers have found that echinacea contains a tumor inhibiting compound. This compound is an oncolytic lipid-soluble hydrocarbon. This particular substance which is found in the essential oil of echinacea, has shown its ability to inhibit lymphocytic leukemia and other types of cancers.

One theory concerning this activity is that it probably does not involve creating a cytotoxic effect directly on cancer cells, but rather stimulates the action of anti-cancer cells such as natrual killer cells already present in the body.

The fact that echinacea inhibits the enzyme, hyaluronidase may also be a factor. The same type of mechanism that breaks down the protective barrier around cells so that disease microbes can enter is thought to occur in the initial stages of tumor formation. Because echinacea prevents the formation of hyaluronidase, it may play a role in preventing the development of certain types of cancer.[16]

## Allergies and Echinacea

German research has demonstrated echinacea's ability to treat certain allergic reactions.[17] It may be the cortisone-like activity of echinacea which accounts for its anti-inflammatory action. In the case of allergic reactions, the immuno-suppressive action of echinacea kicks in.

An allergy occurs when the immune system becomes overly stimulated by the presence of an allergen. Each time that the allergen enters the body an allergic response is initiated. Echinacea can temper this cascade of symptoms by stabilizing mast cells, which are responsible for the histamine release that creates havoc with our bodies.

The fact that echinacea actually suppresses the immune system is nothing less than remarkable. This herb might be referred to as "the botanical with a brain." In other words, it can either stimulate or inhibit immune response as determined by the status of the body. Synthetic drugs do not have this ability.

## Healing Stimulation by Echinacea

Because echinacea has antiseptic properties, it can be used both internally and externally to heal conditions such as bed sores, boils, burns, ulcers and wounds of any kind. The inulin Echinacin B content of echinacea extracted from the rhizome gives echinacea its wound healing properties. It also accelerates the production of granulomatous tissue which is necessary for tissue healing in the body. [18]

Russian studies have shown that echinacea also helps to stimulate healing in wounds and prevents blood clotting.[19]

## Chronic Fatigue Syndrome and Echinacea

Because echinacea contains the polysaccharides inulin and echinacin it may be helpful in fighting stubborn viral infections such as chronic fatigue syndrome. Anytime the immune system becomes compromised due to exhaustion, allergies, or depression, viral and bacterial invasion can occur. The chemical compounds contained in echinacea promote improved resistance to all septic or infectious conditions.[20]

## Prostate Disorders and Echinacea

Echinacea is believed to be one of the best herbs in the treatment of enlarged prostate glands or other prostate disorders.[21] Its anti-inflammatory properties are believed to help decrease swelling and irritation. Tests on mice have shown that using echinacea to control inflammatory responses has resulted in a decrease in edema or swelling.

## Weight Loss and Echinacea

When combined with chickweed, echinacea has been used to promote weight loss.[22] Scientifically, there is a lack of data to explain this particular effect.

## Skin Damage and Echinacea

Any type of skin damage, whether caused by injury or infection can be treated with echinacea. One of the major actions of this herb is its ability to inhibit a specific enzyme that weakens connective tissue cells when they are exposed to certain microorganisms. This enzyme is called hyaluronidase.[23] Whenever skin cells have been compromised by infectious organisms, echinacea can help prevent the spread of infection and speed the healing of the skin by preventing the breakdown of skin tissue at the cellular level. The anti-hyaluronidase action of echinacea, especially when applied as a poultice, can significantly prevent infection and enhance healing in burns, cuts, and abrasions.

In addition, topical applications of echinacea are valuable in treating snake and insect bites. German research suggests that echinacea extracts and salves can benefit a variety of inflammatory skin conditions including psoriasis, eczema, and herpes.[24]

## Yeast Infections and Echinacea

Yeast infections are caused by an fungus called Candida albicans. This particular organism has been the subject of intense interest, research and controversy over the last several years. Standard medical therapies for yeast infections usually involve the use of antibiotics and antifungal drugs which can, in themselves, compromise the immune system. In laboratory tests using control groups, subjects who received echinacea were compared to those who took standard antifungal treatments. In these cases, better results were obtained with the echinacea.[25]

It is the polysaccharides contained in echinacea which seem to enhance the resistance of the immune system against the Candida fungus. This finding again stresses that echinacea may have important therapeutic applications for anyone who is in a weakened state and susceptible to opportunistic infections.[26]

Echinacea in both external and internal forms can be used to treat yeast infections. It has been suggested that anyone who has recurring yeast infections should consider adding echinacea extract to their repertoire of health supplements.

## Inflammation, Arthritis and Echinacea

Some laboratory tests have demonstrated that echinacea has certain anti-inflammatory properties which can help prevent or decrease the inflammation and swelling typically found in arthritis sufferers. Unlike the inflammatory response of the body to infections, the chronic inflammation of joint diseases such as arthritis is not desireable. In these cases, echinacea can help to inhibit chronic inflammation. Its effect is considered equal to approximately half of that resulting from steroid drugs like cortisone in arthritic patients.[27]

Apparently, echinacea contains a specific factor which prevents inflammation and swelling when observed in certain laboratory tests. This particular tonic action may be quite helpful for people who suffer from chronic arthritis. Arthritis symptoms result from an immune response which creates inflammation in the joints. As is the case with allergies, when arthritis is present, echinacea inhibits the inflammatory action of the immune system.

It is interesting to note that another component of echinacea actually boosts the inflammatory response when it is appropriate. For this reason, wounds respond well to echinacea.

Steroids are commonly prescribed for inflammatory diseases such as arthritis. Because steroid drugs have so many negative side-effects, echinacea may prove to be an invaluable treatment for improper immune system reactions that cause conditions like arthritis.

## HIV and Echinacea

At this writing, the possible role of echinacea on HIV has not been established. While some preliminary studies look promising, much more research is needed to determine whether or not echinacea's stimulation of immune function will benefit AIDS patients.

# SUMMARY

Echinacea can be used for a number of different disorders, however, its primary strength is its ability to prevent and treat infections. It can be considered a blood purifier which helps to neutralize the effects of venoms and chemical toxins in the blood and as a vital immune system booster. It has been used for everything from yeast infections to ulcers, to tuberculosis and gangrene.

Echinacea can be thought of as a natural antibiotic and is especially beneficial for colds, flu, and sore throats. Combining echinacea with myrrh is thought to potentiate its action.

Echinacea can actually suppress immune function when that function is not desireable as seen in allergies and arthritis. In these conditions, it acts as a natural anti-inflammatory. The safety of echinacea has been shown in a number of laboratory tests using oral or intravenous applications of the herb. It has been proven to be virtually non-toxic in doses amounting to many times the human therapeutic dose.[27] Whether you pronounce echinacea with a soft or hard "ch" sound does not change the fact that it is one of the most usable plants in the herb kingdom and is applicable in the fields of both homeopathy and allopathic medicine.

# SPECIFIC ACTIONS ASSOCIATED WITH ECHINACEA

- Echinacea works like an antibiotic by simulating the immune system and has none of the side effects of antibiotics.
- This herb is especially effective in treating sore throat, earaches, colds, and viral and glandular infections.
- The action of echinacea blocks the receptor site of viruses on the surface of cell membranes which prevents the cell from becoming infected.
- Echinacea helps the body rid itself of waste material and toxins. It can help reduce edema and water retention.
- By activating and potentiating the immune system, echinacea can help treat infectious disease through its natural anti-viral, and antibiotic properties.
- Studies suggest that echinacea may help to prevent certain types of cancer.
- Echinacea has the ability to suppress the immune system when desireable. This makes it valuable in the treatment of inflammatory diseases and allergic reactions.
- Echinacea is an effective blood cleanser.
- It can help relieve pain and swelling.
- As a wash, it can treat skin disorders such as eczema, burns, psoriasis, herpes, canker sores and abscesses.
- Echinacea stimulates the adrenal cortex, which naturally stimulates the release of cortisol, an anti-inflammatory agent.

## Combinations that Enhance Echinacea

- echinacea, alfalfa, bayberry, capsicum, comfrey, ginger, ginseng, lobelia and myrrh
- echinacea poke root, golden seal and capsicum
- echinacea and elcampane
- echinacea and myrrh
- echinacea and yarrow
- echinacea and golden seal
- echinacea and ginseng
- echinacea and licorice
- echinacea and astragalus
- echinacea, lapachok, comfrey and horsetail

## Primary Applications of Echinacea

- acne
- arthritis
- bites/stings
- blood disorders
- boils
- burns
- bronchitis
- canker sores
- chronic fatigue syndrome
- colds
- congestion
- contagious diseases
- diptheria
- ear infections
- eczema
- fevers
- herpes
- gangrene

- glandular disorders
- gums
- infections (viral and bacterial)
- inflammation
- influenza
- immune system disorders
- kidney infections
- lymph gland dysfunction
- mouth sores
- mucus
- peritonitis
- prostate disorders
- psoriasis
- rheumatism
- skin disorders
- sore throat
- tonsillitis
- wounds

## Secondary Applications

- allergies
- bronchitis
- cancer
- digestion
- diphtheria
- eczema
- fevers
- gangrene
- gingivitis
- staph infections
- strep infections
- syphilis
- typhoid fever
- yeast infections

# ENDNOTES

[1]Claire Kowalchik and William H. Hylton, Editors, *Rodale's Illustrated Encyclopedia.* (Emmaus, Pennsylvania: Rodale Press, 1987), 176.

[2]Louise Tenney, "Echinacea", *Today's Herbs.* (Provo, Utah: Woodland Publishing, Vol. XIII, Number 1, 1993), 1.

[3]*Family Guide to Natural Medicine.* (Pleasantville, New York: Reader's Digest, 1993), 303.

[4]Andrew Weil, MD, *Natural Health, Natural Medicine.* (Boston: Houghton Mifflin Company, 1990) 236.

[5]Gary Gillum, Editor, "Echinacea" *Today's Herbs.* (Provo, Utah: Woodland Books, Vol. I Issue 11, July, 1981), 1.

[6]Penelope Ody, *The Complete Medicinal Herbal.* (New York: Dorling-Kindersley, 1993), 53.

[7]Michael Murray, ND and Joseph Pizzorno, ND, *Encyclopedia of Natural Medicine.* (Rocklin, California: Prima Publishing, 1991), 58.

[8]V.H. Wagner and A. Proksch., "Immunostimulatory Drugs of Fungi and Higher Plants", *Economic Medicinal Plant Research.* (1985), 1, 113-53.

[9]Louise Tenney, *The Encyclopedia of Natural Remedies.* (Pleasant Grove, Utah: Woodland Publishing, 1995), 50.

[10]Ibid.

[11]Daniel B. Mowrey, *The Scientific Validation of Herbs.* (New Canaan, Connecticut: Keats Publishing, 1986), 119.

[12]Murray, 59.

[13]Michael T. Murray, N.D.. *The Healing Power of Herbs.* (Rocklin, California: Prima Publishing, 1995), 100.

[14]J. Mose, "Effect of Echinacin on Phagocytosis and Natural Killer Cells", *Med. Welt.* (1983), 34, 1,463-7.

[15]M. Stimple, A. Proksch, H. Wagner, et al., "Macrophage Activation and Induction of Macrophage Cytotoxicity by Purified Polysaccharide Fractions From the Plant Echinacea Purpurea",

*Infection Immunity.* (1984), 46, 845-9.

[16]Mowrey, 119.

[17]Ibid., 250

[18]Ibid., 119

[19]Ibid.

[20]Ody, 176

[21]Velma J. Keith and Monteen Gordon, *The How To Herb Book.* (Pleasant Grove, Utah: Mayfield Publishing, 1983), 29.

[22]Louise Tenney, *Today's Herbal Health.* (Pleasant Grove, Utah: Woodland Publishing, 1992), 60.

[23]Daniel B. Mowrey, Ph.D., *Echinacea.* (New Canaan, Connecticut: Keats Publishing, 1995), 31.

[24]Ibid., 33.

[25]Ibid., 41.

[26]C. Steinmuller, J. Roesler, E. Grottrup, G. Franke, H. Wagner and Matthes Lohmann, "Polysacharides Isolated From Plant Cell Cultures of Echinacea Purpurea Enhance the Resistance of Immunosupproes Mice Against Systemic Infections with Candida Albicans and Listeria Monicytogens," *Int-J-Immunpharmacol.* 1993, July: 15(5): 605-14.

[27]Ibid., 43.

[28]U. Mengs, C. Clare and J. Poiley, "Toxicity of Echinacea Purpurea. Acute, Subacute and Genotoxicity Studies, *Arzneimittelforschung.* 1991, Oct. 41(10): 1076-81.

# ADDITIONAL REFERENCES

Becker, V. H. *Against snakebites and influenza: use and components of echinacea angustifolia and e. purpurea.*. Deutsche Apotheker Zeitung, 122 (45), 1982, 2020-2323.

Buesing, K.H. *Inhibition of hyaluronidase by echinacin.* Arzneimittel-Forschung. 2, 1952, 467-469.

Foster, S. Echinacea, *Nature's Immune Enhancer.* Healing Arts Press, Rochester, VT., 1991.

Hobbs, C. *The Echinacea Handbook.* Eclectic Medical Publications, Portland, Oregon, 1989.

Keller, H. *Recovery of active agents from aqueous extracts of the species of echinacea.* Chemie Gruenenthal G.M.B.H., Ger. Oct. 11, 1956, 950, 674.

Kuhn, O. *Echinacea and Phagocytosis.* Arzneimittel-Forxchung, 3, 1953, 194-200.

McGregor R.L. *The taxonomy of the genus Echinacea (Compositae).* Univ. Kansas Sci. Bull. 48, 1968, 113-142.